Table of Contents

Introduction 1

About This Guide 3

Part 1: Basic Fundamentals of Face Mask 5

    Why urge homemade fabric face masks now? 7

    What the CDC says about homemade face masks today? 8

    Some Mask Rules: 9

    Is it possible for everyone to wear a mask? 10

Part 2: Types of masks 13

    Scientific approach to make your own homemade mask 14

    Choosing a material 16

Part 3: DIY Your Mask At Home 21

    No-sew options if you cannot sew 21

    How to make a face mask with Grocery Bag 21

    How to Make a No-Sew Face Mask with Bandana, Scarf, or Handkerchief 31

    Steps to Make It 31

    Alternatives to a Bandana, Scarf, or Handkerchief 35

    Alternatives to Rubber Bands 35

    Caring for Your Mask 36

    How to Make a No-Sew Face Mask with a T-shirt 37

Part 4: Sewn Cloth Face Covering 41

   How to make a face mask with Cotton Fabric 41

      The right way to wear a face covering or cloth face mask 45

   Appropriate use of non-medical mask or face covering 45

      Non-medical face masks or face coverings should: ... 45

      Non-medical masks or face coverings should not: 46

      Can you reuse your face mask? 47

Part 5: CHILD SIZE FACE MASK 49

   YOUR SUPPLIES 49

   How to Get Kids to Wear a Mask 54

      Be Honest (But Not Scary) 55

      Get Your Kids Involved in the Design 55

      Turn the Mask into a Costume 56

      Make a Mask for a Buddy 56

      Do a Trial Run 56

      Offer a Reward 57

      Turn it Into a Game 57

      How to Use a Face Mask Safely 58

      Preparing to Wear the Mask 59

      Putting the Mask On 59

      Taking the Mask Off 60

      Keep in mind 61

Part 6: When to use it, Why and Where 63

   When to wear a mask at home 63

Whether you are wearing a face covering or not, the CDC still recommends that you: 64

How to put a mask on and take one off 65

Why masks matter more for this virus 65

What precautions can I take when grocery shopping? 66

What precautions can I take when unpacking my groceries?... 68

Homemade masks may help protect others from you 69

Homemade masks may help protect you 71

Limitations 73

Introduction

A mask is not as good as the wearer and is not a substitution for physical distancing and proper hand hygiene. Everyone should have their own masks to use in public in a better environment to assist to prevent the infection from spreading secretly, and the CDC is currently considering suggesting that everybody use masks in public, not just people with indications.

Sadly, masks are a little difficult to get around right now, so purchasing masks limits the availability for health professionals who are in need of them. Even if the CDC does not issue a new guideline, it is possible that someone who cares about a suffering loved one will have at least a couple so they can sanitize one while carrying another.

Searching for the strategies to bring home your own face mask? If YES, then here is a full guide to continue with much less expenditures and no experience. When learning about face masks for VIRUS protection, there are usually three types: fabric homemade face mask, surgical mask, and respirator N95. Once you begin to make face masks, make sure you understand the difference between the styles, how they can assist to prevent VIRUS from spreading and the components you require. I understand you must have concerns, so I am breaking down what you have to learn about creating and wearing from hand-crafted masks to no-sew covers, and even bandanas tied to your ears through hair ties.

About This Guide

This guide is all about the **Homemade Face Mask** and it is unique from all of the others. The way the guideline is designed makes it easier to find the solution you are looking for. Go ahead and click the Guide to see for yourself. Nice bold headings direct your eyes to only the section you like, and you do not have to read the whole text for a quick response. This guide offers an exhaustive description of all facets of DIY your mask at home. Need details about how to get started? Here is the description too. So, place this tutorial up on your bookcase in a prominent spot. We are confident you will go back to that again and again.

Part 1: Basic Fundamentals of Face Mask

In its suggestion the CDC stresses the use of "face coverings," not simply "face masks." So, what is the distinction? Every fabric that protects the nose and lips, like a scarf or bandana wrapped across the forehead, may be a face mask. A face mask relates to a more particular design, which typically includes padding which is more suited to the nose, lips, and head, as if using ear bands.

Mask guidelines will quickly get confused, as not all masks are completely equal. Other than handmade caps, even medical practitioners, who are prone to the maximum VIRUS levels, are in severe scarcity. Sometimes, they are hard to match properly. The CDC does not suggest them for overall use, for these purposes. The CDC also does not suggest surgical masks to the public at large, due to a shortage. Such masks do not fit against the face but have nonwoven layers of polypropylene and are immune to moisture. Homemade cloth masks are the safest for general population.

Fabric masks which are officially approved by the CDC for common use. Fabric masks often let air in through the edges but neglect non-woven sheets that disperse moisture. They just hinder about 2 percent of ventilation in.

Except the other way around, what? When a mask holder coughs or snores, the membrane may be adequate to absorb a lot of the original nastiness jet — even if there are holes in the cloth or along the edges. The goal of the new mask experiments was to answer this: whether handmade fabric masks did a great job of virus confinement. Yet their downside is that DIY face masks are easily accessible and by chatting, coughing, spitting, and snoring can help alleviate the large particles that are expelled.

Why urge homemade fabric face masks now?

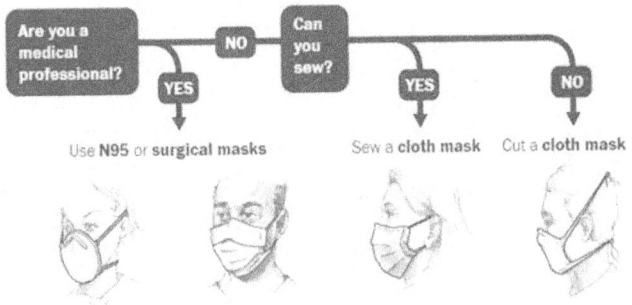

The CDC has suggested facial masks for months for those who were suspected to be or reported to be infected with VIRUS, as well as for emergency care staff. There are also evidence suggesting there might be some value of using a DIY mask of busy areas such as the store, as opposed to no face shield. Physical detachment and handwashing are also of utmost importance.

All persons wearing the masks may provide a level of membrane defense against respiratory droplets which are snorted or sneezed around them. Initial reports suggest that, after an infected person has left an environment, the virus will survive in particles in the air for up to one to three hours. Wrapping your skin helps keep any particles from hitting the air and contaminating others.

What the CDC says about homemade face masks today?

The most significant lesson from the CDC's warning is that it is a "voluntary global health initiative" to hide your face as you leave home and does not override established measures such as home self-quarantine, physical distancing, and extensive sanitizing.

In the terms of the CDC it "prescribes wearing cloth face covers in public places where other physical distancing steps (e.g. grocery stores and pharmacies) are difficult to maintain, particularly in areas with substantial community-based distribution.

CDC should not search for medical or surgical masks on its own and keep N95 respiratory masks to nurses and doctors, alternatively opting for fundamental clothing or fabric face masks that can be cleaned and recycled. The organization actually considered homemade face masks a last-ditch effort in clinics and hospitals.

Even a clear mask is very helpful in catching particles from your sneezes and cough. A recent survey has been reported to exhale into a giant tube, filled of multiple viral infections (influenza, rhinovirus, and a more moderate form of virus). Occasionally they didn't cover their noses and mouths; other hours they used a plain, not-particularly-fit mask.

The contaminated men, without the masks, exhaled infectious droplets and pollutants, small particles that lingered in the soil, about Thirty percent of the time they were examined. This covered almost Hundred per cent of virus particles but some of the aerosol particles while the sick people wore a mask.

Looking at all the findings together, we found that the bulk of virus-laden respiratory droplets and some virus-laden aerosols could be avoided.

Some Mask Rules:

Do not buy the surgical masks and keep them. Medical professionals are already facing a crippling supply shortage, and we should not use surgical masks that might be used for sick patients and health professionals.

Do not place a face mask on children under the age of 2—or anyone who has trouble breathing or may not be able to take away the mask themselves.

Do not cover a mask by the area of its lips. Seize it by the ties. Rinse your hands when you touch it.

Is it possible for everyone to wear a mask?

At the moment the World Health Organization (WHO) states that just two categories of people can wear face masks, those that are:

- Infected and showing signs
- administering for people who probably suspects to have this virus
- This says the healthcare staff will have surgical masks secured.

For the public at large, masks are not suggested, because:

- They may be affected by coughs and snores from other individuals, or when they are placed on or removed

- Regular hand laundering and social distances are much more productive. They might offer a false sense of security

Part 2: Types of masks

N95 respirator masks: These masks fit securely onto the face and have the best filtration capacity, trapping 95 per cent of 0.3 micron or bigger particles. An N95 mask prevents health care staff who comes into contact with large doses of the virus when treating and conducting numerous patient treatment services. That standard of security is not required for the majority of us, and these masks can only be used for medical care staff.

Medical masks: Such are still in demand and cannot be used by emergency staff. Often referred to as surgical masks or operation masks, these masks are square shaped garments which come with flexible ear loops. Medical masks are constructed from paper-like nonwoven stuff and are often offered to a patient waiting for a physician to see. Relative to the N95 mask, a medical mask removes between Sixty to Eighty percent of particles and also covers "large-particle droplets, splashes, sprays or splatters that may comprise pathogens," according to both the Food and Drug Administration.

Homemade fabric masks: The Centers for Disease Control and Protection advises that, when we are in public places, we shield our faces with a blanket or DIY cotton mask. Homemade masks differ in efficacy depends entirely on the cloth used, texture and design.

21 people have made their own masks out of T-shirts from another survey, and analysts compared the DIY masks to the surgical masks. "All masks considerably decreased the number of pathogens ejected by volunteers," the researchers wrote, even though the surgical masks were safer. Homemade masks have been found in group experiments to provide some security against viral infections.

Scientific approach to make your own homemade mask

Keep in mind that any facial covering is safer than no face cover. Although certain individuals use air filters and ventilation bags to play with DIY masks, the average individual does not require that degree of security if you exercise physical distancing and leave the house only for the crucial. Given that there is so much variety in materials, a light check is the safest recommendation. Keep the cloth or mask against the light, to see how much light falls. The stricter the weave, the less light you are going to see and the more preservation you get. However, check the cloth over your face to ensure that you can indeed breathe through this one.

Researchers have been studying everyday products because of a lack of masks to see how well they could fit in a handmade mask. They also related the volume and scale of the diluted molecules to the normal used by surgical masks — 0.3 microns. Checking two surfaces of materials use around 1-micron particles though. An analysis shows that the 0.3-micron check is an awesome quality, the 1-micron test will also be important to assist people to have a choice about mask substances.

"In 1-micron droplets / aerosols there are possibly a lot of further viruses than in 0.3-micron droplets / aerosols." "And even though a mask absorbs just 20 percent of 0.3-micron droplets / aerosols in thickness, it usually performs best with 1-micron droplets / aerosols, synthetic biology."

Here is a glance at some of the daily products that have been tested for homemade masks. You can check out so much in this book, What's the Right Material for Mask?

Choosing a material

T-shirts: Many of us have an old T-shirt which we could turn into a no-sew mask. It is one of the best common materials to use, but there is a great deal of variation in how well T-shirt clothing works in laboratory studies. A single sheet of an old cotton T-shirt caught twenty per cent down to 0.3 microns of molecules. It trapped Fifty per cent up to 1 micron of molecules. Two T-shirt sheets that trapped about Seventy per cent of molecules down to 1 micron.

Cotton quilting fabric: For its toughness this is the strong-thread-count synthetic fabric favored by quilters. Safety masks constructed from quilting cloth rivaled the filtration capacity of surgical masks in tests.

Tea towels: The tea towels are a common source of material for masks. Researchers have found that coating good in contrast to a 1-micron molecule scale medical mask. The creators of the analysis did not take care of the mark. The towel utilized was not a terry fabric, but a finely knit array of absorbent tea towels.

Pillowcases: Pillowcases are a great choice for sewers that have no other fabric. Two pieces of pillowcase fabric evaluated near to the effectiveness of the surgical mask at the 1-micron specification, but in a research, four layers of 600-thread-count pillowcase stuff were needed to attain the 0.3-micron conventional amount of security.

Flannel pajamas: One of the finest evaluated was a two-layer mask of flannel and silk which paralleled the reliability of a surgical mask.

Coffee filters and paper towels: For additional protection, the C.D.C. recommends putting a coffee filter into your mask. It is discovered that three coffee filters have made breathing difficult. Including a sheet of paper towel among two sheets of cloth will keep the handmade mask quite effective and a single paper towel filter twenty-three per cent of 0.3 microns and two paper towels filter thirty-three per cent. Our handmade T-shirt mask was applied with a paper towel.

Scarves and bandannas: You cannot top a mask or bandanna to shield your face when it comes to user kindness. Yet bandannas are small, that do not provide enough security, even rolled over four days. Scarves may be safer, but they can be warm and heavy. Both are safer than almost zero.

Optimally, the face mask of the bandana will blend snugly with your face and there are no spaces between your face and the mask. But you do need to make it easy, so you will not be able to change or re just the mask. If you should contact the front of the mask, washing your hands with sanitizer Lysol, or warm water.

Filters and vacuum bags: Researchers who are seeking to identify successful solutions for medical personnel have hacked down air filter layers and checked HEPA vacuum bags. Both can operate very well, but there are major disadvantages to both. When cutting air filters can unleash fibers that may be harmful to inhale, so if used in a mask the filter stuff should be wedged between layers of heavy cotton fabric. Vacuum bags are fine filters, but they are not so breathable. Besides, some vacuum bag brands can include fiberglass so do not use it to hide your face.

Part 3: DIY Your Mask At Home

No-sew options if you cannot sew

If when it comes to sewing you do not know where to start, there is a no-sew face mask choice. You should use tissue glue and an iron rather than stitching the cloth together. The iron is being used to weld together tissue and glue. You will also use the iron to make pleats for a stronger mask in the cloth.

When you do not have either of those items, you can use a scarf and some hair ties or elastic bands to create a face mask easily — once, this is for individual purposes.

How to make a face mask with Grocery Bag

Let us make this very clear: Masks are not assured to guard you from VIRUS, no matter how efficient.

This guide is an easy project for those with no sewing machine. Although cotton is requested in several ventures. There is no suggestion that it is better or bad than other textiles — it is cozier, and people want to keep it on hand. According to the theories of experts about the hydrophilic (water-loving) properties of the cotton masks that lead to increased levels of respiratory infection. Usage of a plastic hydrophobic substance identical (but not identical) to that used in surgical masks. And many individuals in their own home do get it right.

Tools

- Needle and thread
- Scissors
- Ruler
- Clothing iron
- Sewing or safety pins
- Permanent marker
- (Optional) Seam ripper

Materials

1. Medium non-woven polypropylene reusable grocery bag
2. Pipe cleaners (or plastic-coated twist ties)
3. (Optional) 60 inches of ribbon, between ½ and 1 inch wide

Instructions

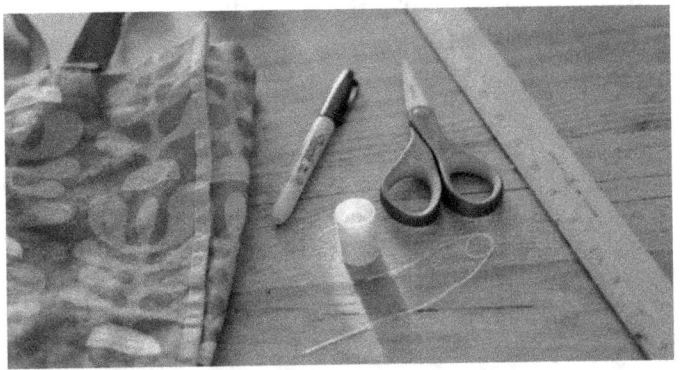

1. Wash the reusable grocery bag.

Caution: We explicitly suggest a reusable, non-woven polypropylene shopping bag (NWPP for short), not a reusable plastic one. It may sound stupid, but you have to breathe via the mask. Keep away from insulation packs (these normally have some inside foil material) or protective plastic lined containers, too.

Note: Pick the bag with the biggest handles you can get if you can. If you can use them as braces for the mask this design would be simpler. If the loops are not long sufficient, we will clarify how to construct ribbon belts.

2. Cut the sides off the grocery bag so the material lays flat. Do not cut off the handles.

3. Cut the material into two sheets. If your bag has a seam at the bottom, cut it like you did the side seams. You will get two clean sheets of NWPP, each with its own handle.

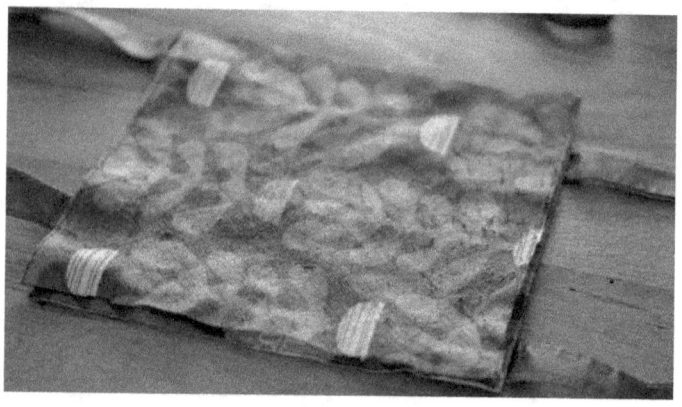

4. Measure and cut one sheet. Evaluate the top edge of the bag with the scale to reach the middle. Place your permanent marker on it. Using that as a point of reference, calculate back 4 1/2 inches and trace again against each stick. Calculate 9 inches from each point and make parallel vertical lines of cutting. Link the down lines. You must have a 9-by-9-inch square at the highest level with the clamp, with a completed (sewn) edge.

Note: When the handle is too big to fit within the square you have weighed, skipping over **(step 8)** and then use ribbon substitute **(step 9)** is the easiest option.

5. Repeat Step 4 on the other sheet of material.

6. Sew the mask's side seams. Put one layer on the wrong side (the former interior of the bag) and pull half an inch of content from the rim of the handle opposite. Iron the fold to put on low pressure. Sew it from the bottom then a quarter inch. Position the other layer on the right-hand side (the previous exterior of the bag) and fold it in half an inch like all the other layer, iron it and stitch it a quarter of an inch from the bottom.

Caution: Polypropylene is a plastic sort of thing. The use of an environment with high temperature will melt it, destroy your task and, most definitely, your iron. If there is no setting for "poly" then choose the smallest setting (usually silk) and every it marginally if the fold is not set.

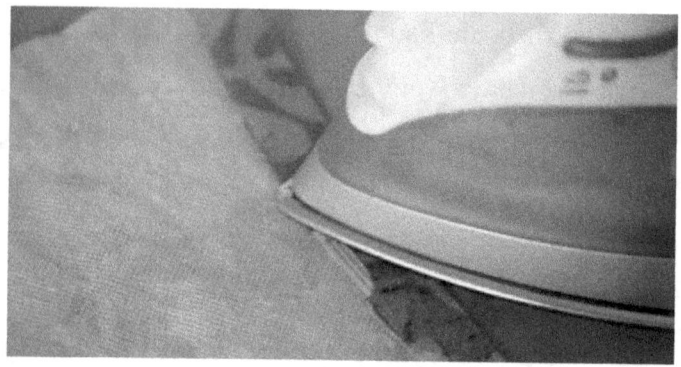

7. Place the sheets together. Your mask will have tissue on two layers. Position one of the layers on the work surface and approach the handle to the left. Position the other one over it, the handle confronting to the right. Pin on the spot.

Note: We suggest looking the same way on the illustrated side of the covers, because the back of the mask is a different color to the face. Davies claims this will better ensure that you do not misplace the mask, with the dirty side toward your mouth and nose, by mistake.

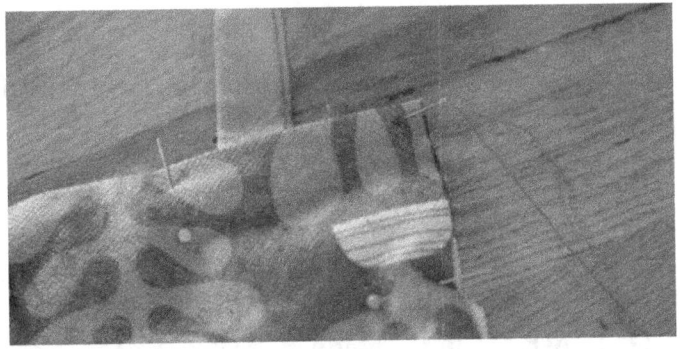

8. Make the head ties. Cover in half the handles and cut them in the middle. Keep the mask fixed over your face with loops sticking out from the bottom, and make sure the handles are long enough just to cover the back of your head with at least 4 inches to spare.

9. (Optional) Make straps out of ribbon. If your bag's handles are not long enough to even be belts, you'll have to build your own. Start taking the NWPP layers off the handles or use a seam ripper to clean them. Place the mask in the middle of your face and use the measuring tape to calculate the length of each brace — each brace should be sufficiently long to extend from the side of your neck to the back of your head and clip behind this one securely. Split the badges and pin them wherever the handles were.

Placing your mask on check the fit. If the ribbon size is correct, dual your thread and sew the pieces on the wrong side of the sheets into place.

10. Sew the sheets together. Double your thread and sew all of the corners around.

11. Finish the bottom edge. Create a half-inch fold at the base as you did in Step 6, and iron it. Sew it shuttered from the rim by a quarter of an inch.

12. Make the adjustable noseband. Cover half an inch over the upper lip, then weld this again. Wrap or twist the pipe cleaners together and cut them to the exact width as the mask. Wrap in to break them at their ends. Inside fold tuck the metal bonds and pin the bend over them. Then stitch the fold underneath and on the sides of the links to secure them in position.

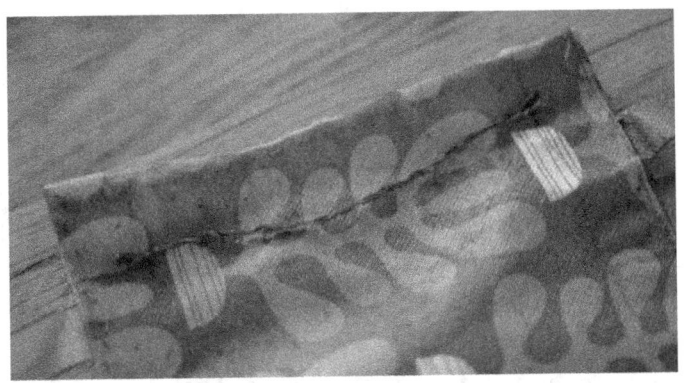

13. Make three folds to pleat the mask for expansion. Pleats should be about 1 1/2 "wide on the outside, half an inch broad on the inside, and overlapping to the nose band. If it benefits, trace the lines on the cloth, folded the rows and then iron them. Wrap this into place by sewing a quarter inch from the bottom of both ends. This time, twice the normal stitch back to ensure good plough edge.

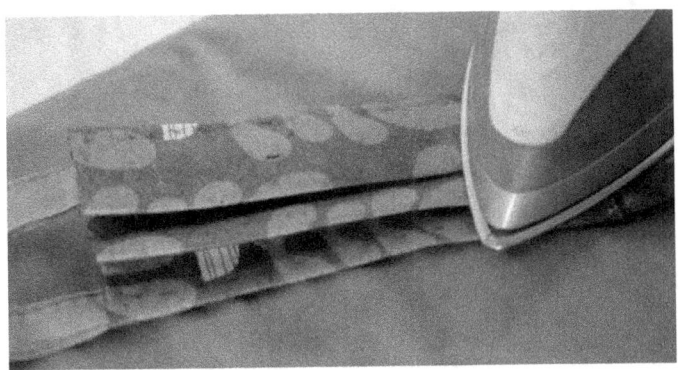

14. Sterilize your mask Immerse the mask in hot water for 10 minutes until first use. Undo the move between various uses.

Remembering one face mask simply is just not enough. Also make sure you bring glasses or sunglasses to shield your eyes and have never open the section covering your lips. Disinfect it when finished, let it dry thoroughly (in the sun if you have access) to avoid the bacteria from growing and then place the mask in a safe, waterproof, resealable container.

How to Make a No-Sew Face Mask with Bandana, Scarf, or Handkerchief

It is easier to make a no-sew face mask than you would imagine, which is a perfect option if you can't sew or don't have the right stuff. A no-sew mask is a fast task everyone can do — you don't have to be especially crafty or have needle and thread expertise. The biggest news is it takes just about five minutes to make it. Remember, you won't need to go out for materials, because this face mask guide just uses only things that you already have at home. At the end of this article we have mentioned possible tactical changes, just in case you don't have any of the recommended products.

Materials

- 1 Bandana, scarf, or handkerchief
- 2 Rubber bands

Steps to Make It

Only a few things you'll need to create your face mask no-sew. The bandana, scarf, or handkerchief has to be at least 20 inches by 20 inches, so covering your nose and mouth is massive enough.

1. Prepare Your Fabric

Use bandana, t-shirt, or other cloth that you want to use. Keep putting your cloth tight on the board, the shaped side experiencing the table and the back side confronting you.

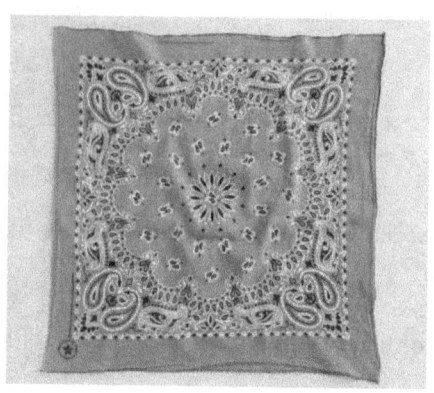

2. Make the First and Second Folds

Pick the top surface of the cloth and flip it over so that it meets the bandana center. Do that for the bottom half and folded up the cloth until it comes to the middle of the bandana, reaching the leading edge you folds down.

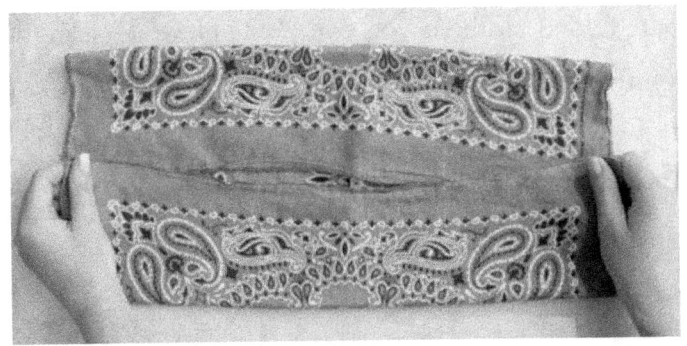

3. Repeat the Folds

Finish two further bulges by lining up at the top to the center and the underside to the middle. It will make a few pleats which will facilitate the mask to suit your face better.

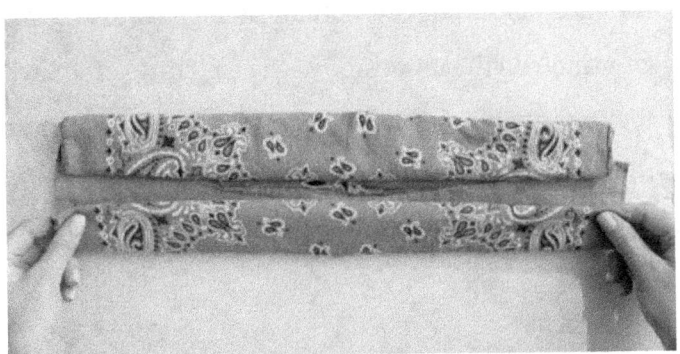

4. Fold the Ends of the Fabric

Wrap the right and left sides into the middle of the cloth rectangle. Now you'll have a shorter rectangle of folded cloth so you can put a piece of string on either side.

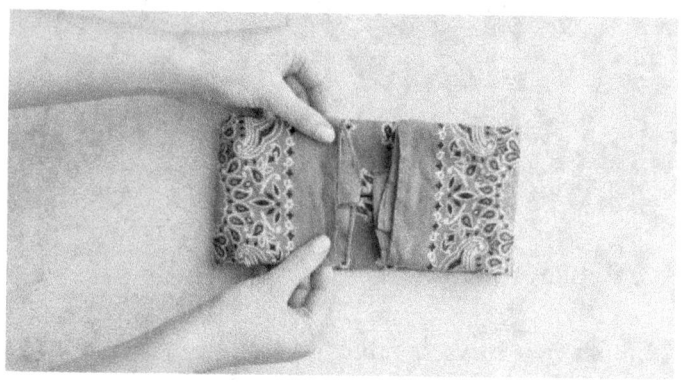

5. Slide on the Rubber Bands

Take a group of rubber and slide over one end of the rolled-up cloth, having left a few inches to the other. Continue on the other side of the rolled-up cloth, with the other rubber band. If you want you can curl one of those folds inside another to protect the fabric better, but that's not essential.

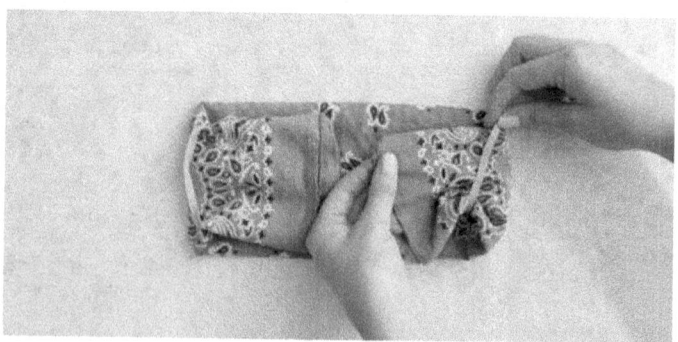

6. Finish Your No-Sew Face Mask

The side which faces you will be the mask's behind. Now, it's prepared to just use! Take the mask to your mouth to use and place the elastic bands around your ears to keep it secured. The mask would protect both lips and nose.

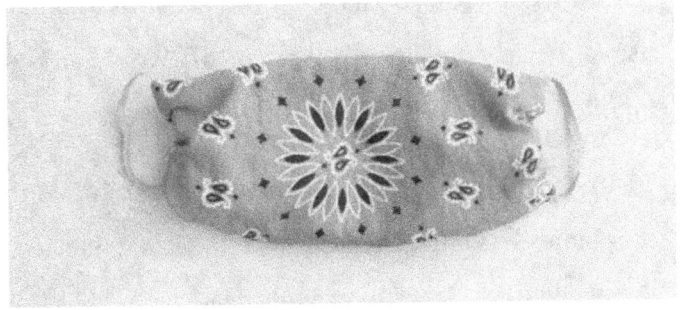

Alternatives to a Bandana, Scarf, or Handkerchief

You should cut an outdated piece of clothing if you don't have any of these things at. Textile cloth works likewise in a squeeze jersey garment from an old work. To make this no-sew mask, you will have to cut slits of fabric which is 20 "x 20."

Alternatives to Rubber Bands

If you don't have accessible rubber bands, there are a couple of other choices. When you have ties to the hair they're going to fit well. Only be sure they've got a lot of width on them.

There are several other choices if you don't have elastic bands or hair ties. You may trim an elastic loop from a set of pantyhose, tights, or leggings. You should take off part of the nylon cuff or the stretched part of the sole if you have an old pair of socks, just use it. Nearly any length you cut off would fit well about 1/2

Just note that whatever you are using to remove the hair bands has to be as stretchy as these bands will be the aspect that aligns over your head.

Caring for Your Mask

Such masks are wonderful for being usable and so easier to take care of. Only remove the elastic bands and clean the fabric just as you'd have a regular item of clothing. After every use it's suggested that you clean the cloth masks. To wrap your mask, keep reposting this tutorial, so you can dress up it once again.

How to Make a No-Sew Face Mask with a T-shirt

Steps

1. If you've got an old T-shirt, so you should transform it back into a face mask.

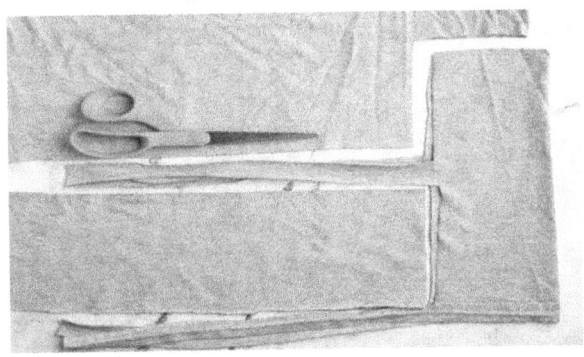

2. Cut this type out of a t-shirt beginning at a folded bottom. The two sections of rope should be about 12" long by 1" high, and the rectangle at the folding edge should be about 4" high by 14" large. When opened, the rectangle in the middle will be spanning 8" by 14".

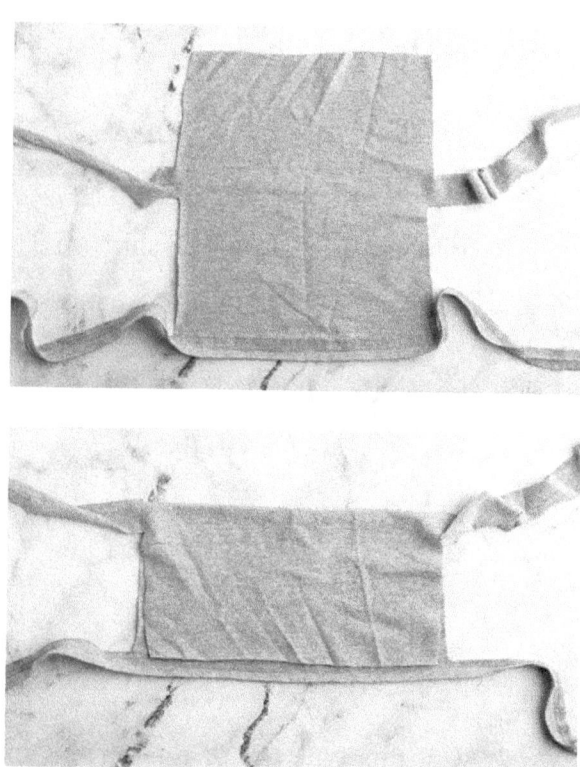

3. Place the slice of cut out and pull the top half down over the lower half. (That will show you two sheets of fabric on the main component of the mask.) After you've rendered that flip, there'll be four links at the four edges.

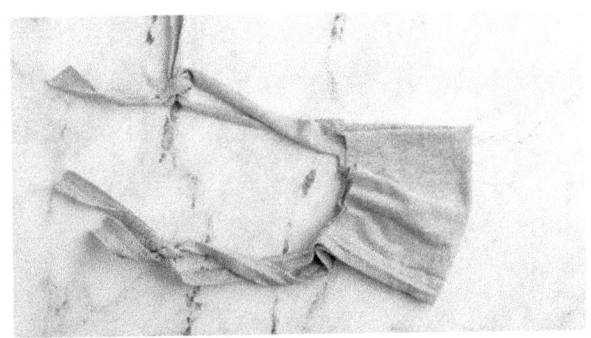

4. Knead the buckles behind head and behind the neck to dress up the mask. To change the fitting, you can put both braces behind the head

Part 4: Sewn Cloth Face Covering

How to make a face mask with Cotton Fabric

Materials

- Two 10"x6" rectangles of cotton fabric
- Two 6" pieces of elastic (or rubber bands, string, cloth strips, or hair ties)
- Needle and thread (or bobby pin)
- Scissors
- Sewing machine

Tutorial

1. Break out two 10-by-6-inch cotton print rectangles. Using closely knit cloth, such as cloth sheeting or quilting thread. T-shirt fabric is about to function in a small pot. Place the two rectangles; knit the mask as if it were just a single piece of fabric.

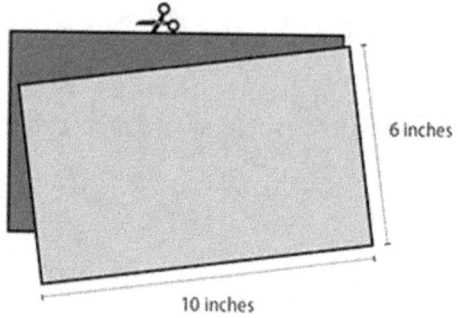

2. Fold in 1⁄4 inch and spread over most of the long sides. After which wrap over 1⁄2 inch over most of the short sides of the dual layer of cloth and sew down.

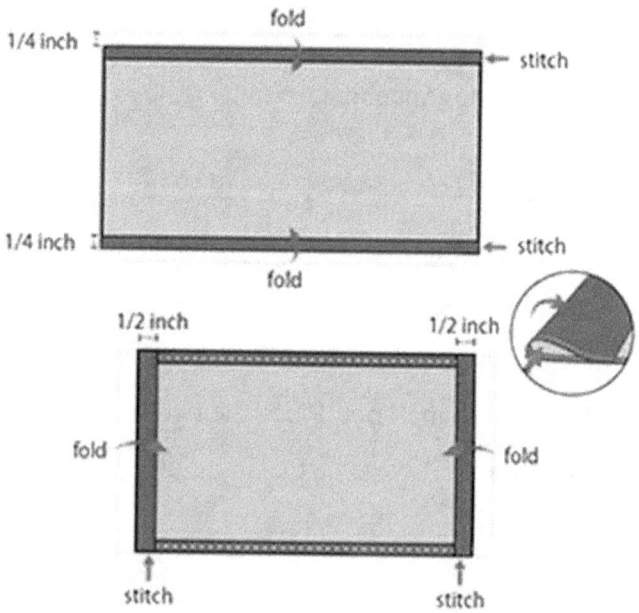

The top image shows the two bits of rectangular fabric which are piled on top of each other and meet on both directions. The triangle, standing straight, is placed so that the top and bottom of the triangle are the two ten-inch sides, while the left and right sides of the rectangle are the two six-inch sides. The top image shows the two long sides of the rectangle of fabric being folded over and sewn into place to create a one-fourth inch margin around the whole width of the rectangular top and bottom. The below image shows the two narrow sides of the rectangle of fabric being flipped over and stapled in order to create a one-half inch fringe over the whole range of the right and left side of the facial protection.

3. Pull a 1/8 "long rubber 6-inch length through to the wider fringe on either side of the mask. Those are going to be the ear cords. To loop it through using a wide needle or bobby pin. Bind the tight ends.

Aren't elastic? Using elastic head bands or hair chains. You can keep the links bigger if you just have rope, and bind the mask around your back.

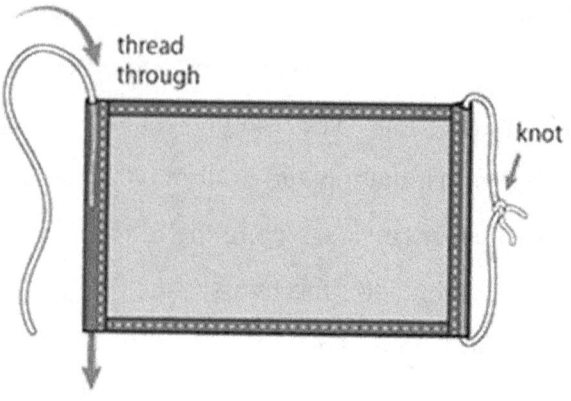

Two six-inch sections of rubber or rope are woven through the free, half-inch hems formed on the rectangle's left and right sides. Instead, the rope or string's two ends are bound together in such a band.

4. Push softly onto the rubber to tuck the loops within the hem. Pick the mask sides on the rubber and change the mask to suit the face. Instead tie the rubber tightly in order to prevent it sliding.

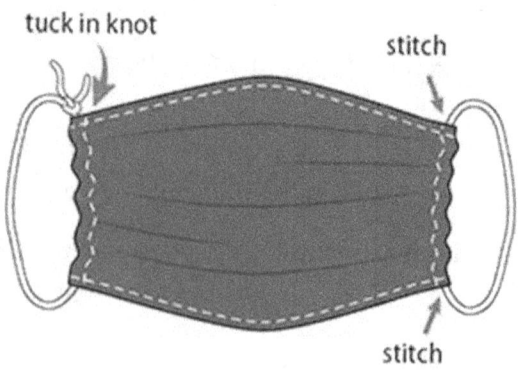

The right way to wear a face covering or cloth face mask

The first and most critical thing is to cover both of your nose and mouth, ensuring that the face mask will work under your jaw. When you're in a busy market, the shielding would be less comfortable if you take it from your face, like talking with someone. It is safer, for instance, to change your wrapping before you leave your house, instead of standing in line at the store. Check on why fit really is so critical.

Appropriate use of non-medical mask or face covering

An individual using a non-medical mask or face shield will decrease the spreading of his or her own contagious respiratory particles when properly attired.

Non-medical face masks or face coverings should:

1. Enable easy breathing
2. mesh safely to the head with ties or ear loops
3. to sustain their texture after washing and drying

4. to be altered as quickly as possible if humid or dirty

5. be comfortable and do not require regular modification

6. at least 2 layers of interwoven product fabric (such as cotton or linen)

7. be huge enough just to be completely and easily cover the nose and mouth

Some masks often have a pocket to hold a paper towel or coffee filter which can be disposed of for added advantage.

Non-medical masks or face coverings should not:

1. Be associated with other

2. compromised vision or conflict with activities

3. put on kids under the age of 2 years

4. composed of synthetic or other non-breathable materials

5. covered with adhesive or other unsafe items

6. made entirely of items that quickly break apart, such as tissues

7. put on someone unable to extract them without help or someone with difficulty breathing

Can you reuse your face mask?

Homemade masks and cotton fabric coatings are machine washable. Medical-grade masks are usually single-use but the extreme lack of N95 masks makes surgical limitations a must in many hospital conditions.

Part 5: CHILD SIZE FACE MASK

I set out to create mask model Child Size Face for you. This is really simple, and it takes only 10 minutes to do it, basically. For your and the children of your loved ones, you should make up a couple of these. This Face Mask for Child Size measures about 5"x 7". For various ages I'll send different measurements.

YOUR SUPPLIES

For ages 4-12- You require two strips of fabric measuring 5" x 7" and 2 pieces of 6" thick, 1/8th "rubber. If you are unable to obtain thin rubber, you should cut wider ones. Or if you can't seem to find some rubber, you should use long cords to attach them backwards.

For ages 2-4- You require two pieces of fabric measuring 4" x 6" and 2 pieces of 5" thick, 1/8th "elastic.

When your child has a large nose, you may choose to use rubber for further.

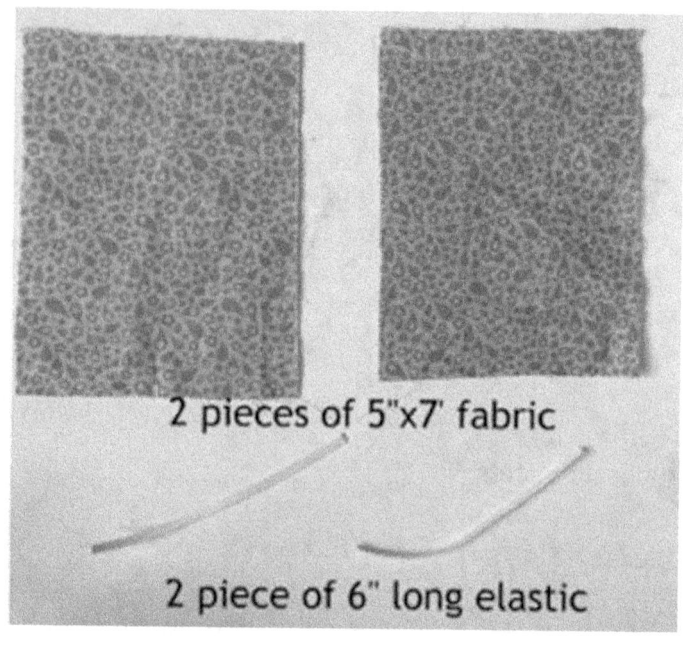

2 pieces of 5"x7' fabric

2 piece of 6" long elastic

LET'S START SEWING

1. Pin elastic around 1/2" from small front side edges of a fabric.

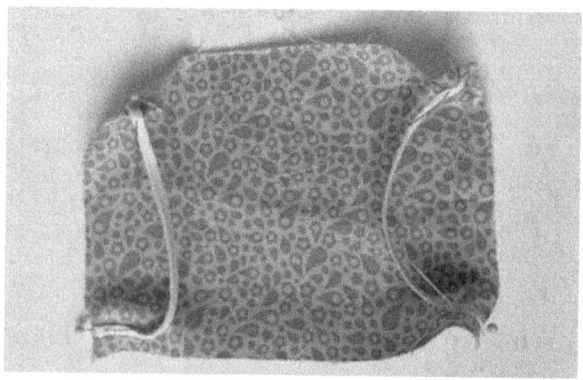

2. Then put the other piece of fabric face down on the right-hand side, and tie it all over.

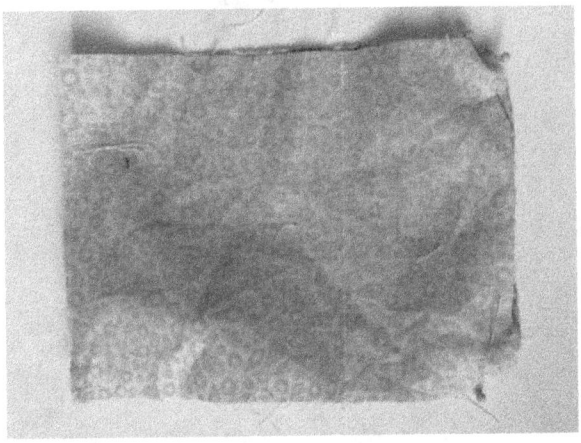

3. Sew the two parts of cloth all over linked. It can be difficult when you have the rubber corners so go slow. Left around 2" free, so that you can transform it inwards.

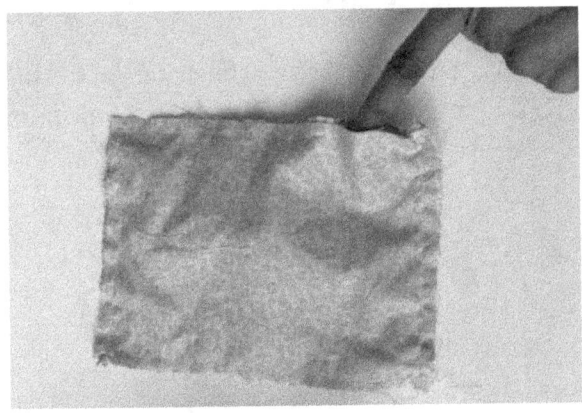

4. Turn inside. Wrap the gap down, then sealed the top sew.

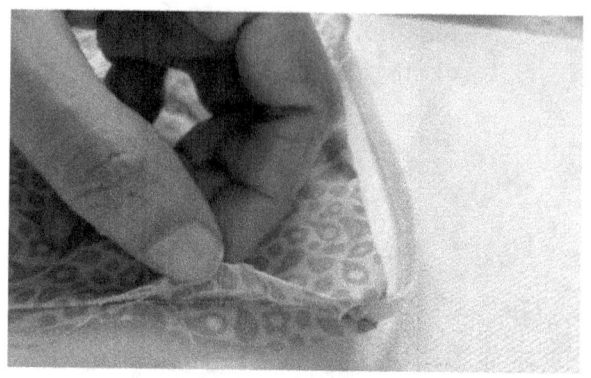

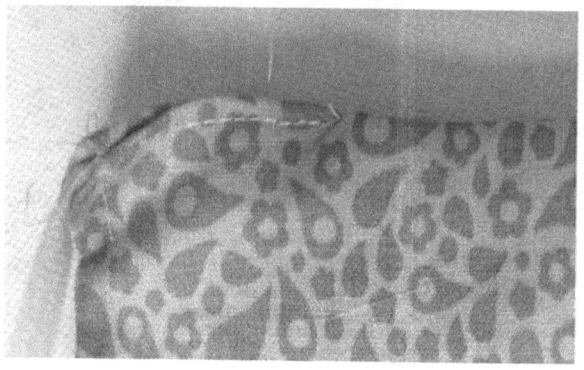

5. Then, do two sheets in the mask's side middle. The pleats are approximately 1" each.

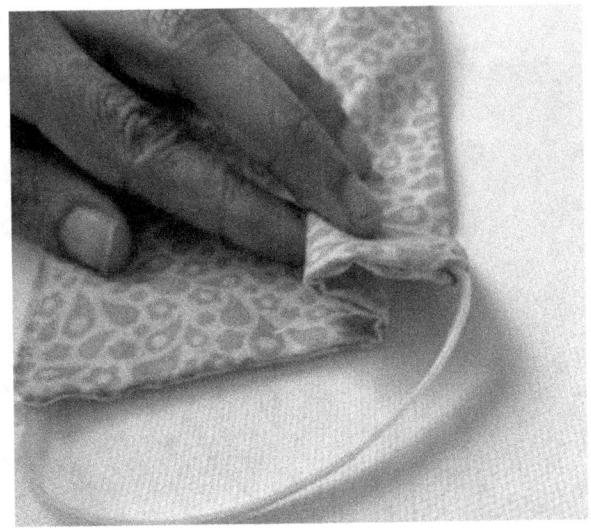

6. Place the folds and tie the ends.

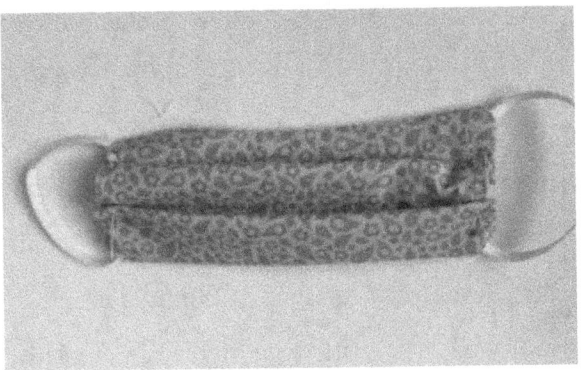

7. That is, it! You are done.

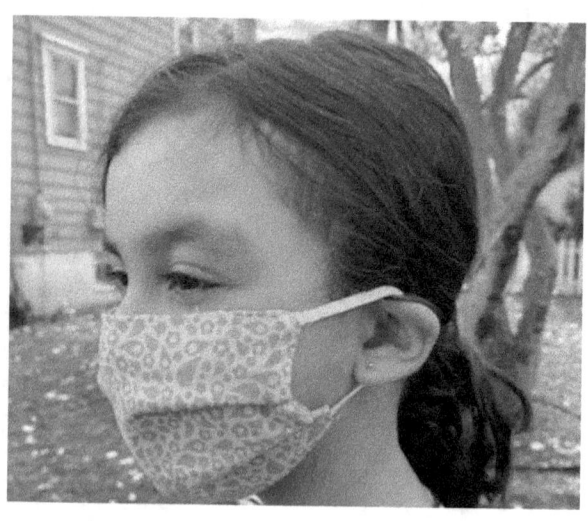

How to Get Kids to Wear a Mask

The safest choice in shelter-in-place and remain-at-home directives is to keep children at home with the other member of the family instead of taking them out. Overall, certain evidence suggests that children are not only likely to become carriers for the disease, they are also at danger of being sick. But when you really have no option but to bring your kids with you, you must have a mask on face.

Here are some suggestions to make the process go a little smoother

Be Honest (But Not Scary)

No matter how old your child is, be frank about why masks are necessary. You do not have to go into any details, and you should keep things age-appropriate so be transparent about the virus for your children.

Clarify to them that wearing a mask enables to protect the people around them. Avoid the temptation of dramatizing the circumstance or revealing more detail than is required. The idea of wearing a mask is then seen as an excuse to convey altruism and sympathy.

Get Your Kids Involved in the Design

One approach to get the children to buy into the notion of wearing a mask is to include them in the cycle of layout. Enable them to pick the pattern they want to use, such as an old T-shirt or a pillowcase featuring their beloved character in the cartoon. Just a simple white shirt or bed sheet they can put on can fit with textile paint. The trick to getting the fabric chosen for the mask.

Turn the Mask into a Costume

If you make a decision to use fabric paint on your kid's mask, assist them transform it into an animal or persona. To make a pup, small cat, or rabbit, it is simple, for example, to paint a mouth and whiskers on the mask. Mix that with some Halloween leftover eyes and you can notice your kids simply cannot wait to use their masks.

Make a Mask for a Buddy

Any kids may have a better risk of wearing a mask if their "buddy" wears one too. So, if your kid has an absolute favorite stuffed animal, an Old granny they're taking anywhere, or another beloved toy, make a mask for them too. And when you head out, they will come along with their partner as long as they have their mask too.

Do a Trial Run

For most kids wearing a mask is a unique experience. Yeah, the first couple of times the kids wear a mask, they can say it's itchy or they can't relax. Most kids aren't going to enjoy the thought of wearing a mask.

Check out the mask at home for this purpose. Let your kid wear it for 30 minutes. Exercise carefully putting it on and not removing it until it's mounted. Afterwards, explore how it feels to wear it for your family. And make modifications to the mask if necessary while also checking that it suits correctly.

Offer a Reward

Often children react favorably to what they're scared to do because they recognize there's a payoff at the end. As a consequence, you will inspire your children to wear their masks and give them something that will look forward to when they get home. For example, they might be receiving a badge for their poster, an ice cream cookie, or even an extra hour of TV to comply with the rules when out in public. You know what your child is inspired by so pick appropriately.

Turn it Into a Game

Other way to get your children inspired to wear a mask is to make it into a challenge. Creating a game out of wearing masks much like the "no talking challenge" or the "who can go the maximum without blinking" challenge. Have everybody start with 10 points, for example. They lose one point every time somebody moves their mask to change it. The one who has the most skill points wins game by the time you arrive home.

How to Use a Face Mask Safely

It's incredibly necessary to use a fabric mask properly. Otherwise you and your kids face the risk of potentially spreading diseases to yourself and others. In fact, the CDC advises that cotton face coverings will not be used for infants below two years of age. They can also not be used by someone who has difficulty breathing, is asleep or otherwise is incapacitated.

If your child is older than two years and relatively well, if you have to go out, it is usually appropriate for them to wear a mask. When you've cleaned the mask of your kid and it's prepared to go, here are few crucial measures to put the mask securely and successfully on:

Preparing to Wear the Mask

Clarify to your kids that it is time to start putting on their masks

Note that they could not contact the masks until they're on or removing them without permissions

Give sufficient time for conversation and attempt not to hurry your kid through the procedure, particularly if it's their first to wear a mask outside

Wash the kid's hands with soap or sanitizer before they contact the mask.

Putting the Mask On

- Pick up the mask by ties or clips with washed hands and properly attach it to your baby's face

- Making sure that the mask fits easily so that your baby still can breathe easily

- Change the cloth around the nose bridge to make it fit tightly (some people feel that holding your child's glasses or even sunglasses over the mask's edge lets her remain in place, but this is not needed).

- Be sure your kids are confident with their masks and warn them that they shouldn't contact it and leave it in place

- Clean your hand carefully, taking into account that you touched the mask and your baby's face

Taking the Mask Off

- Wash your hands until removing the mask and let your kid do the same.

- Note that the kids should not cover their face even though the mask has been taken away.

- Removing the mask through ties or belts

- Place the mask directly in the washer or in a plastic container.

- Wash the mask in a washing machine and make it dry in a drier.

Keep in mind

You should be washing your hands before and after each time you treat your face masks with your fabric. Furthermore, fabric face masks can never be used a second time before they are cleaned.

As well as being filthy from the saliva of your infant, the masks possibly contain pathogens and other pollutants. Keeping the mask on again without cleaning it just raises the risk of infection in your kid. In reality, a study published in the Lancet showed that the virus could live for at least one day on fabric and for up to seven days on surgical masks.

Part 6: When to use it, Why and Where

The suggestion is to wear a face mask in public places at all times, so we do not know who has the infection and who does not. Wearing a mask, particularly though you are indoors, is still more environmentally conscious. According to several authorities, outdoor activity, with or without a mask, remains relatively healthy. Research teams warned that little is known about heavy breathing and how it impacts viral proliferation during aerobic exercise. When someone tugs the mask off to reveal the nostrils. This can make the mask much less efficient when it comes to germ protection.

When to wear a mask at home

In the house, a mask is only required if somebody is sick. The patient should be limited to a single space with little or restricted interaction with the rest of the family (including pets) and can have, if feasible, a single toilet. All sufferer and caretaker will wear a mask when they came into contact.

Whether you are wearing a face covering or not, the CDC still recommends that you:

- **Wash your hands regularly.** Using soap and water for about 20 seconds, then wash them. If you cannot wash your hands, hand sanitizer is permissible to be used.

- **Hide your face** with a towel or the inside of your forearm while sneezing.

- **Stop touching your face**, since you can convey the virus in your throat from your hands.

- **Remain at home**, apart from important visits outside, such as visits to the supermarket or doctor's appointments. Of location, this is also called sheltering.

- **Experience distancing** physically by remaining at least 6 ft away from others. The White House also advises limiting 10 or more meetings which should be easy because you are sitting at home.

- **Wash and decontaminate regularly** hit surfaces daily.

How to put a mask on and take one off

- Clean your hands just first.

- Do not access the mask's cloth part — that is basically the germ barrier, so you do not want to disperse the germs it has captured.

- Use the ear knots or ties to protect and take away your mask. The coverage area will go down under your chin from above your nose bridge and extend to your ears around midway or more.

- Pull the links and loops so they align against your face as snugly as feasible. If there are pleats in your mask, the tucked side will be flat.

Why masks matter more for this virus

To begin with, it is a new virus which indicates that our immune systems have not had it before. It is different from the flu, from which many of us have some safety, either because of significant exposure to influenza-related viruses or because we have been shot. One of the greatest concerns is that there is no virus safety for health staff, who get screened to remain healthy through flu season.

It is also worth noting that the flu season occurs over many months. virus has spread much faster, infecting an abundant number of patients — and leading to tens of thousands of cases — in a matter of month.

An additional twenty five percent of virus patients feel completely normal and do not know whether they are sick and may be infectious. So, what are we to guess? You may well have been one of them! For this purpose, you must wear a mask to shield us from your concealed pathogens.

What precautions can I take when grocery shopping?

It is spread mainly by virus-containing granules, or through viral particles floating in the air. The virus can be effectively breathed in and can also distributed when a human hit a surface, or it is important to note that the flu season takes place over several months. virus has progressed even further, contaminating a large number of people — and resulting in hundreds of thousands of cases of — within a month.

An extra 25 percent of people with virus feel absolutely regular, and do not know that they are ill and may be contagious. And when are we to conjecture? You could have been one of them! To this end, you have to wear a mask to protect us from your secret microbes. An entity that carries the virus and then contacts your lips, face, or eyes. There is no existing evidence of a transmission of the virus by food.

Health measures enable you to prevent virus respiration or contact an infected area and contact your nose.

Keep at least 6 feet of space between yourself and other shopkeepers in the grocery store. Wash the frequently touched surfaces with hot water and soap such as grocery carts or basketball handles. End up having your face touched. Having to wear a cloth mask serves to warn you not to cover your skin which can also serve to prevent infection transmission.

Using hand sanitizer prior departure from store. Wash your hands the moment you return inside.

Restrict the visits to the grocery store if you are older than 65 or at higher risk for whatever cause. Ask a friend or roommate to pick up groceries and keep them outside your house. See whether your grocery store is offering special hours for older people or those with situations underlining them. Or have shipped supermarkets to your house.

What precautions can I take when unpacking my groceries?

Recent research has shown that the VIRUS could survive for up to 72 hours on materials or objects. This means that the virus on the surface of the grocery store should be denatured over the course of time after foodstuffs have been packed away. Try cleaning the outside areas or cleaning them with a sanitizer if you intend to use the goods within 72 hours. It will not infect the entire content of sealed bags.

Washing your hands with soap and water for at least 20 seconds, after unwrapping your groceries. Clean the surface areas you place on while unwrapping them with household cleaning products.

And that is when eating fruits and veggies thoroughly wash with water. And washing your hands before eating some meal you have taken home from the grocery store lately.

Homemade masks may help protect others from you

Homemade face masks cannot be able to eliminate any molecule and are not expected to protect you from contracting the virus, although under certain cases they may support. The extreme lack of N95 masks, which enables to deter the acquisition of virus by medical practitioners such as doctors and nurses, has indicated that ordinary citizens required a substitute to effectively stop the spread.

Using a fabric face mask while you're with people will help trap big particles that you could expel with a coughing, sneeze, or inadvertently released saliva (e.g., through speaking), which could delay the transfer to others if you don't realize you're ill. "These kinds of masks are not designed to protect the user but to prevent him from accidental exposure — in situation you are a virus symptomless carrier.

The only thing you can really do to keep virus from advancing is to clean your hands regularly for at least 20 seconds with warm water and soap. If none is accessible, using a hand sanitizer with an alcohol base of at least 60 per cent.

You can also perform the following parameters:

- Stay at home
- Keeping a 2-meter physical distance from others to shield you. If you cannot sustain physical space, try wearing a non-medical mask or a handmade face covering
- To prevent exposing your ears, lips, nose, or eyes

It has not been proved to shield the person who wears a handmade face covering / non-medical mask in the group and is not a replacement for physical distancing and washing hands. However, even though you have no signs, it could be an extra precaution taken to defend those around you. This would be helpful for brief periods of time where it is not possible to separate physically in urban spaces, such as when searching for food or using mass transport.

Homemade masks may help protect you

While we know that even a standard mask does a fairly better job of shielding the world from your outgoing pathogens, experts believe there's more variability in how well homemade masks could shield you from unspecified pathogens, based on the fit and reliability of the content used.

But the thing is, if you do practice physical distancing and cleaning your face, you do not need an extremely efficient mask. And if you use a cloth of good filtration capacity — like two layers of thick cotton or flannel — and wearing the mask appropriately, you are through the odds of virus avoidance.

The fact of the matter is that you reduce your risk of becoming sick when you start practicing physical distancing, washing your hands, and wearing a mask in those times when you just have to leave the apartment.

Limitations

Non-medical masks are not regarded as potent in obstructing tiny particles as the hard-to-get N95 respirator masks required by the medical profession.

All of this leakage in homemade fabric masks is why public health experts usually do not assume that wearing a mask hinders anyone from catching a virus which is already hovering around in the atmosphere. Flow of air takes the less resistant direction. When viral particles are in the area, they have an easy route around a cloth shield of their own making. And in the specific instance of a handmade cloth mask, people who wear might well waft in tiny sufficient particles to float right through the fabric.

Homemade masks are not medical equipment and as surgical masks and respirators are not governed. Their usage presents a range of restrictions:

- They have not been checked in compliance with recognized guidelines,
- The materials are not the same as those used in surgical masks or respirators,

- The ridges of which are not devised to form a barrier around the nose and mouth that may not offer full protection from virus-sized particles

- That can be hard to breathe and may stop you from getting the reaction